The Health Benefits of Thyroid Metabolism

Strengthen and Save Your Thyroid Glands

Dr. Cass Ingram

Knowledge House Publishers

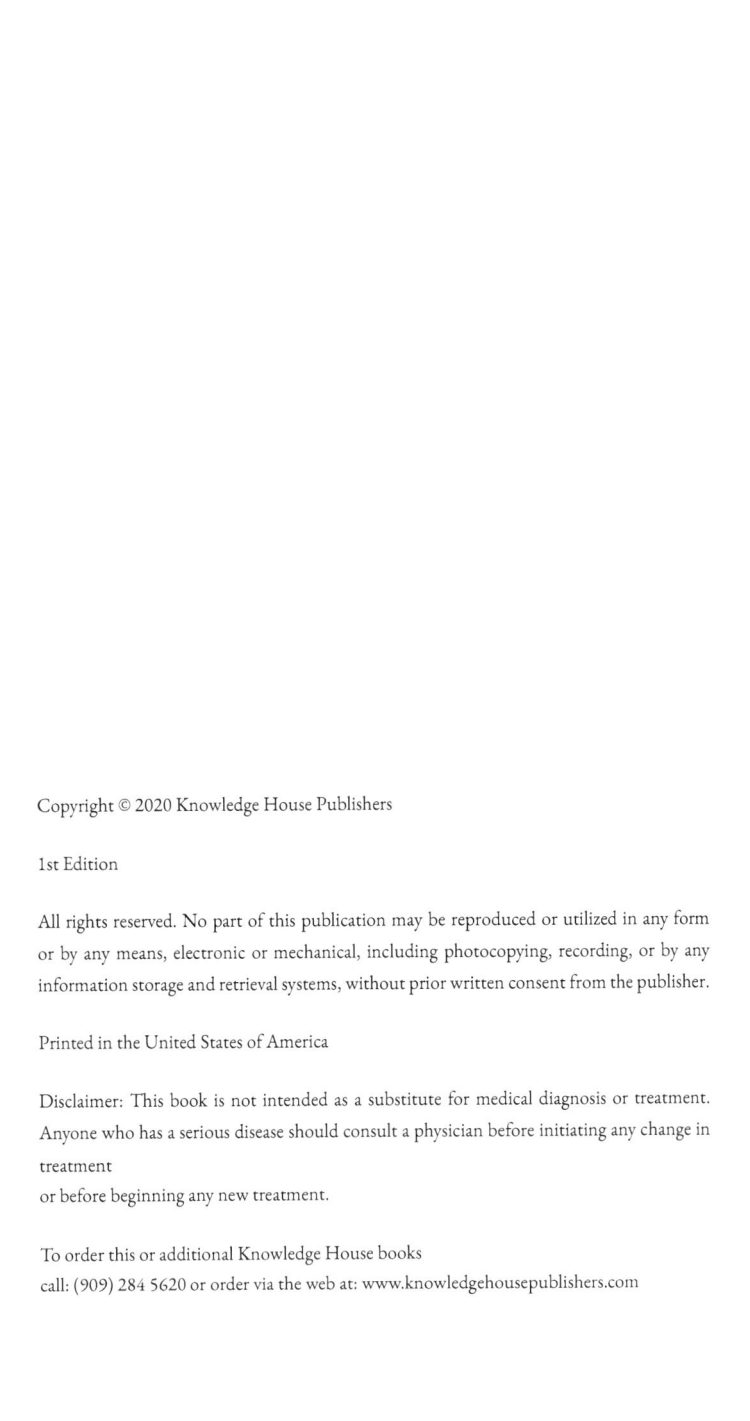

Copyright © 2020 Knowledge House Publishers

1st Edition

All rights reserved. No part of this publication may be reproduced or utilized in any form or by any means, electronic or mechanical, including photocopying, recording, or by any information storage and retrieval systems, without prior written consent from the publisher.

Printed in the United States of America

Disclaimer: This book is not intended as a substitute for medical diagnosis or treatment. Anyone who has a serious disease should consult a physician before initiating any change in treatment
or before beginning any new treatment.

To order this or additional Knowledge House books
call: (909) 284 5620 or order via the web at: www.knowledgehousepublishers.com

Contents

1. Introduction — 1
2. The Thyroid Type in Review — 5
3. Diet and Nutrition — 17
4. Weathering the Storm — 25
5. Thyroid Self-Test — 29
6. Conclusion — 41
7. Bibliography — 49

About the Author — 50

Chapter One

Introduction

There is a novel group of organs in the body that act as chemical factories. Their purpose is to produce substances with signaling power, delivering messages of intelligent instruction to all cells. It is a wireless network, where the active factors operate through the circulation and have direct and irresistible powers over the body. These chemicals are the hormones, and they are produced by a network of organs, known as the endocrine glands. The hormones are chemical messengers, their purpose being to create the necessary communication lines. Hormones essentially instruct the genetics of all cells and organs to do the body's bidding. Importantly, they represent the most powerful substances produced by our bodies and exert that authority in the tiniest of dosages, mere micrograms or less. They have a profound influence upon the internal chemistry, structure, and function. The major glands that exert this control are the thyroid, adrenals, pituitary, and gonads.

These and other glands are the major controlling force for overall health. Circulation, mental function, digestion, skin function, and immunity are all under their authority. Perhaps the main area is the metabolism, which they almost exclusively control. This includes how well an individual absorbs and processes food. The shape of the body, various fat distribution patterns, and finger length are hormone-dependent issues. Actually, from that shape plus signs and symptoms it is possible to determine the hormone status.

The hormone system is also related to the nerves. This is through brain structures such as the hypothalamus but also the pituitary. This is control center for the entire endocrine system. Yet, then, it is controlled by the brain itself. Thus, the connection to hormone function with the nerves is direct. This explains the potentially severe impact of psychic stress upon hormonal function.

This book is about the thyroid hormone component, specifically, the thyroid type, although in all cases there is a connection to the other endocrine glands. It is possible to determine the type through a highly accurate method of self-testing. If a person turns out to be a thyroid type, that means there is a lack of function, that is a deficiency. This is critical to determine, as it could make the difference between sound health and the onset of disease. In contrast, a person who lacks the signs and symptoms has by inference an adequately functioning organ. The other main categories are adrenal, pituitary, thyroid-adrenal, and, more rarely, adrenal-thyroid; there are separate pocketbooks that deal with the majority of these. There are also ovarian and male gonadal, although they are not covered here. This booklet will deal with only two, thyroid and thyroid-adrenal.

A lack of thyroid secretions leads to tell-tale signs and symptoms. Those symptoms are well-known and include exhaustion, especially in the morning, cold intolerance, insomnia, depression, and short-term memory loss, among dozens of others. The physical features easily demonstrate the condition, especially fat distribution, areas of swelling, finger length, shape of the face, overall body shape, hair loss patterns, and other physical features.

Endocrine disorders occur most commonly in females. This is in part a consequence of the strain upon the glands from pregnancy, childbirth, and nursing, which can be considerable. According to W. Engelbach, M.D., in his book Endocrine Medicine in the 1930s the ratio of female to male endocrine disorders was 3:1. Now, it is even higher, as much as 5:1.

Everyone, though, male or female, must know their type. Not knowing may put the individual at risk. After all, the thyroid gland controls the metabolism in all cells, including those of the heart, arteries, brain, liver, skin, and kidneys. Obviously, then, knowing for certain the pattern aids a person greatly, and this would largely be in relation to disease prevention. It also assists, monumentally so, in dealing with any health concern: in healing and recovery. Now, through the body type program a person no longer operates via guesswork. This is crucial, because a lack of a deliberate, scientific approach can prove disastrous. Undiagnosed thyroid disorders can result in heart disease, strokes, diabetes, and arthritis. Even depression may result as well as skin disorders and sleeping disturbances. Clearly, the endocrine status, when insufficient, determines a person's vulnerabilities. This insufficiency must be dealt with in order to achieve the necessary prevention, it is also critical in order to reverse the dysfunction, all to avoid chronic disease as well as premature death. The point is knowledge is power and through this, it is possible to control the destiny in a positive direction.

The number one killer: a thyroid disorder?

In this state the vulnerability to serious cardiac individual, such as congestive heart failure and heart attacks, is exceedingly high. Broda Barnes, M.D., in *Solved, the Riddle of Illness* proved long ago that regardless of the syndrome all people with heart and circulatory disease have thyroid components. He had found a constellation of people dying from heart disease, especially congestive heart failure, at a young age. Tying this to hypothyroidism he directly halted the death rate through the prescription of thyroid hormone. By taking certain preventive measures, Barnes determined, the heart attack risk, as well as the risk for stroke and congestive heart failure, was essentially eliminated. This is an incredible feat, proving that the thyroid gland controls the most essential of all life processes.

In hypothyroidism the diabetes incidence in is exceptionally high. Both pre-diabetes, that is syndrome X, and the actual disease itself may rapidly develop in the event of the deficiency. There may be a curious connection that is virtually never considered. Thyroid types are vulnerable to fungal overload. If the fungus is not fully cleansed from the body, cancer development is likely. Low thyroid itself acts as a cancer precursor, especially if the TSH is high. It is known that TSH or thyroid stimulating hormone is a carcinogen, which makes sense since it is a genetic or cell growth agitator, Regardless, this vulnerability could be greatly diminished by natural immunotherapy, for instance, the regular intake of oil of wild oregano and the aromatic water of wild oregano.

\

Chapter Two

The Thyroid Type in Review

A butterfly-shaped gland wrapped around windpipe; the thyroid gland is known as the "Master of Metabolism." It exerts and influence over dozens of body functions. This includes decisive power regarding the major organs, including the heart, intestines, and brain. Having a major impact on growth and sexual development, failure to thrive and delayed sexual maturation are typically signs of its dysfunction. It also has a direct power upon the immune system. In this regard it controls body core temperature, which greatly impacts the bone marrow. This is where the majority of blood cells, white or red, are produced. As well, reduced thyroid function has a negative impact upon digestion and elimination, including the production of digestive enzymes, hydrochloric acid, and various intestinal secretions.

Thyroid hormone controls the rate of metabolism or the combustion of fuel in virtually all cells. By combustion is meant the burning of both the food sources of fuel and also oxygen. It is related to intracellular energy production through high levels of activation in the mitochondria. Therefore, the production of the most basic of all energy sources, ATP or adenosine triphosphate, which drives all activity, is a thyroid-based synthesis.

Since the hormone stimulates the metabolism in all cells, a lack of it causes a highly predictable circumstance. This is a full-body slow-down. Weight gain may result, and in the extreme, there is usually an accumulation of substances that lead to a kind of swelling or puffiness. These are the mucopolysaccharides. Loving water, they distort the cells and organs through swelling the body's components—the skin and even the organs. This leads to a potentially life-threatening condition, known as myxedema. A metabolic derangement, myxedema can mild or extreme. It can be recognized as a swelling or thickening in the texture of the skin as well as the shape of the face, arms, legs, and torso. Internally, the brain, heart, and liver mainly are impacted and also swell or thicken. This internal organ damage can rapidly cause a decompensated state, leading to fatality. This demonstrates how crucial are thyroid secretions for the functional operations of the organs.

Let us look at the list of the main symptoms in the thyroid type, being listed for hypothyroidism, as published in medical textbooks:
- fatigue and lethargy
- mental sluggish and depression
- dry, coarse skin
- muscle cramps
- decreased memory, especially short-term
- numbness and tingling
- impaired hearing
- moderate weight gain, like 10 or 20 pounds
- intolerance to cold
- decreased sweating

- generalized joint pain
- coarseness of the voice, loss in women of naturally sweet tone
- hand and finger swelling, also of the face, legs, and arms

This list will give individuals a strong idea of whether or not they fit the category. If a person has at least three of these, it is fairly certain this type applies. Five or more is a virtual guarantee.

Still, people will be confused. Thus, for them, there is a need for absolute conformation. This can be down online through the highly sophisticated, thorough Website, www.ebodytype.com. It can also be achieved through the book The Body Shape Code (formerly The Body Shape Diet, same author). For ease and rapidity, though. the test on the Website is preferable, which is even more thorough than the book as well as more updated. Plus, a person could evaluate the status of the adrenals, pituitary, and possibly gonads to determine what role they contribute. This is because collapse of a gland function is never isolated.

The slowing down of the metabolism is the major issue. No cell or organ that evades the disruption. This includes, as indicated, digestion, elimination, heart function, immune powers, skin health, and mental ability. Even the nerve cells become sluggish, therefore the numbness and tingling as well as, centrally, impaired memory.

One way this slow-down can easily be diagnosed is the body temperature. Thyroid hormone is behind the creation of a normal temperature. Orally, this is 98.6 and about 97.6 in the body core. Anything lower than this is proof of dysfunction. As popularized by Barnes, there is a simple way to rely upon this to tell the exact thyroid status. This is the underarm temperature test. This is how it is done. Place a thermometer at bedside. Upon awakening, do not move or get up. Place the thermometer well into the armpit. Leave for 10 minutes and record. Measure this for 10 days-straight or at least a week and make a chart. Menstruation nullifies the results. A temperature of 97.6 and above indicates normal thyroid function. Below this is abnormal, with significant hypothyroidism falling at 97.0 and lower. If this measures in 95 or 96 degrees, this is a sign of severe sluggish thyroid function.

There is no way the body can operate optimally at a 2- or 3-point temperature drop. This abnormally low status has a great deal to do with the thickening as, essentially, metabolically, the cells become clogged up. A normal or even slightly high body core temperature is needed for keeping the tissues in a fluid state. With this drop the fluid nature of the tissues is lost and the cells become congested.

The temperature test is often more revealing than blood tests. With the blood tests it is usually difficult to impossible to diagnose early cases. By the time it shows up in lowered serum results, some 60% or more of thyroid function may already be lost. A high TSH indicates a near total failure of the organ. Often, there can be a considerably low core temperature, even though the blood tests are normal. Also, low normal serum results should be recognized, as this is usually neglected by medical professionals.

Partly because of these metabolic derangement thyroid types develop a distinctive shape and look. This is the apple shaped body conformation with a thickening. There is, as well, an atypical type, which is watermelon shaped, the long 'Texas' kind. Apple shaped is extremely classic and helps make the assessment easy. It's an upside-down apple, to be exact (see Figure 1). It is the self-test on www.ebodytype.com and also found in the Body Shape Code that will aid in confirming the exact thyroid status. Even so, thyroid types develop a distinctive clear-cut physical feature. Besides the apple shape in the front there are certain patterns to the rear. As a rule, in the thyroid classification a person looks like a virtual half apple, as, typically, the buttocks are flat. This is compared to the pituitary and ovarian types, where they are plumper. The legs have their own look, almost cylindrical or tree-trunk appears, the kind which goes straight up. Laterally, they are flat without considerable cellulite, unlike pituitary persons, who are loaded in this regard. The same is true of ovarian types, who have a fat pad that protrudes out laterally.

Physiology and chemistry

No one really understands the chemistry of the thyroid gland. This is being guessed at, the idea that there are just three key hormones: T3, T4, and calcitonin. Yet, it truly is impossible to know exactly how the gland operates. There exist numerous cofactors that work in unison with the known agents. This is why the crude sources are preferable to the drugs. In cases described by Larsen, endocrinological surgeon from the 1930s, great strides could be made with the opposite approach of standard medicine. This was through relying on a crude, whole food approach where people would reject the aggressive use of surgery and potent drug isolates. The surgery, he found, was particularly disastrous, when such a critical endocrine organ, such as the thyroid and ovaries, was removed. He was in favor of full-spectrum sources, whole glandular material and the consumption of flesh rich in thyroid hormone components. In some cases, there was complete reversal of the pathology with this entirely natural method. In addition to the glandulars grass-fed meat is an optimal choice, while to a lesser degree poultry and seafood provide supportive power. Animal flesh is dense in thyroid hormones, fully lacking in vegetation, kelp and dulse being the main exceptions.

How to treat a thyroid type

Usually, the sluggish thyroid is treated with medication. The main one of concern is Synthroid. How can a synthetic hormone replace the natural production? Yet another is pork-derived thyroid complex, which is isolated T3 and T4. No human can fully comprehend the complexity of the thyroid system. When at all possible, natural, unprocessed supplements would be preferably to man-made drugs. While pork derivatives are natural, they do have challenges. One of these could be contamination with porcine coronavirus, essentially the same as the one infecting the world today. This could wreak havoc and cause the individual to test positive to this infection, even though not being actively contaminated.

The option is crude, whole food sources. One of these is the Body Shape Code thyroid support supplement. Containing thyroid complex from the whole food gland, it provides all the dozens of substances found in the thyroid organ. The exceptions are T3 and T4, which must be taken out by law. Note: it is not so much the danger of these that is the issue but, rather, this law was created by the makers of thyroid hormone, notably Armor Meat Packing, so a monopoly could be maintained. Another medicinal crude source is kelp. It also contains a variety of thyroid-supporting hormones, also pre-hormones, in an entirely natural state. Beware of cheap imitations made from feed-lot based cattle, which is dense in highly noxious GMOs.

Reviewing the thyroid type: signs and symptoms

In the thyroid type the myxedema is a major catastrophe. People can have elements of it, that is it may not be full-blown. The typical case is that the tissues appear unusually thick, even swollen. The contour of the facial bones is often lost. In the extreme the tissues are puffy, leading the fat to a droop or sag. The corners of the eyes droop downward, as do the corners of the mouth. The eyes themselves are typically swollen, where there can be puffiness on the eyelids and around the sockets.

Many thyroid types have a roundish head, yet for others it is square. The main issue are the patterns of swelling, which can be found throughout the face and also neck.

In most cases there is sufficient swelling that the clavicles can't be seen. The abdomen may be protruding, but there is a lack of fat deposition on the lateral thighs and buttocks. This obesity of the abdomen is known as peritoneal fat and represents an increased risk for heart disease as well as diabetes.

The swelling can continue onto the hands, where there is a puffiness all the way to the fingers. This is to such a degree that, in women, they may difficulty removing their rings by the end of the day. Swollen ankles and feet are also common in thyroid types.

In women with thyroid disorders there is usually evidence of other dysfunction, notably that of the ovaries. There may also be a mild- to modest-adrenal gland insufficiency. Doctors have traditionally treated this gland as an isolated organ, giving potent drugs. This is an erroneous approach. The thyroid gland is part of a symphony of endocrine organs. Thus, treating it with isolated or synthetic drugs may temporarily resolve many of the symptoms, but the dilemma is when such potent hormones are taken long-term, imbalances inevitably develop and there may be significant organ damage elsewhere. Even the thyroid gland may suffer from an imbalance, hopelessly repressed due to the overpowering effects of replacement hormone.

True, some individuals have no option but to regularly take thyroid drugs, for example, as a consequence of the surgical removal of this gland or its destruction by radioactive iodine. In such cases individuals are essentially thyroid cripples. They must take the hormone or risk serious consequences. However, for all others the ideal treatment is to create a balanced function, where the thyroid produces its own hormones and where it, therefore, is able to function adequately, without medication. Yet, even in extreme cases proper nutritional and herbal supplement regimen may help normalize the thyroid glands, even, perhaps, without the need for medication. One supplement which always seems to assist in these difficult cases is the wild oregano. This can be taken as the oil, juice-essence, and the whole, crude herb. There full understanding of wild oregano's powerful impact upon the thyroid is still unknown. It is, though, a decent source of iodine and other key minerals such as magnesium and zinc.

Let us revisit the issue of medicine's approach. The delicate balance of this gland and its secretions is demonstrated by the well-known results of taking thyroid drugs. The person may experience nervousness, agitation, sweating, rapid heartbeat, heart rhythm disturbances, chest pain, and possible digestive disorders. The synthetic version, Synthroid, is associated with osteoporosis, that is bone loss. In particular, with toxic reactions to Synthroid cardiac symptoms may predominate; there may be excessive nervousness as well as skipped beats. There can be palpitations and racing heart. It is merely that the intake is greater than can be metabolized. The hormone accumulates, and this agitates the cells. Also, this is only a single hormone, while natural-source thyroid consists of multiple hormones. Thus, the organ system is thrown out of balance through the regular intake of synthetic thyroid hormone.

It has been presumed that deranged thyroid function is due primarily to iodine deficiency. It has also been established that goiter is directly caused by such a deficiency. It was again Larson in his book Why We Are What We Are who takes issue with this. He claims that the blaming of all goiter and/or thyroid conditions on a lack of this substance is fraudulent. Weak secretions of the entire endocrine glands, not merely the thyroid, he established, are the cause of goiter. He defines this further by claiming that it is weakness of the secretions during puberty which is the major factor. Thus, he proposes, if the endocrine glands could be naturally strengthened during this time, the entire problem of sluggish thyroid and/or goiter would be eliminated.

There is a degree of modern proof for this. It is now known that many cases of sluggish thyroid syndrome, as well as goiter, develop in teenagers. For modern youth the body simply cannot cope hormonally with the stress of growth. Nutritional deficiency increases the risk. What's more, the intake of highly processed foods precipitates it. Larson notes that in such teenagers simply nourishing the glands and providing hormonal supplements normalized the function, usually within the year. He gave no iodine. However, his experience has been recently upgraded, that is through a combined approach. This is because there is often even a greater degree of improvement if good nourishment, hormonal support, and natural iodine sources are combined. With such an approach virtually any childhood or teenage thyroid condition can be cured, without medication. Yet, with such an approach Larson proved that the chemical therapy method, giving only one substance, like iodine drops, is ill-advised.

Here is more evidence against the single chemical theory. Iodine can act in a negative way. In some people it may provoke an emergency situation, that is Hashimoto's thyroiditis and also potentially fatal hyperthyroidism. In these conditions and also in some inflammatory goiters it is contraindicated. As proven by Larson the approach should be to overall balance the endocrine system. He noticed that while young girls and teenagers had swollen or distressed thyroid glands, this rarely happened in young teenage boys. In even young children he made the same findings. He describes a family of, ten children, five females and five males. The females all developed swollen thyroids, while no such deformity occurred in the males. This he attributed to the fact that the females had to contend with the menstrual cycle, which places great stress not only on the thyroid but also the ovaries and adrenals. With this stressful dysfunction the stage was set for thyroid collapse, since this gland helps control the menstrual process as well as the food metabolism. By causing these various glands to function in balance Larson cured the thyroid disorders as well as goiters.

Yet, even Larson determined that iodine is critical. It is desperately needed by both the thyroid gland and the ovaries. The ovaries concentrate this mineral, where it stimulates the secretion of female hormones, including estrogen and progesterone. Plus, these glands produce their own iodine-based thyroid-like hormone, diiodotyrosine. Thus, the thyroid and the ovaries work as a unit, and, therefore, any supportive therapy must take this fact into account. Only by normalizing the function of both glands can sluggish thyroid and/or goiter be efficiently cured. In fact, the thyroid-like hormones produced in the ovary have a direct effect upon the thyroid, as well as other female organs such as the breasts and uterus. This is why in order to correct any supposed thyroid disorder the ovaries must also be treated. Thus, as claimed by Larson "goiter is due to endocrine dysfunction."

Weak adrenal glands may play a role in undermining thyroid function. In the case of inflammatory disorders of the thyroid, such as Hashimoto's thyroiditis, Grave's disease, and hyperthyroidism, the primary defect is adrenal. As well, such diseases are associated with infections of both the adrenals and thyroid, primarily by fungi and even tuberculosis. Or, systemic infection may be the main perpetrator, including in hyperthyroidism infestation by worms. Such infections must always be suspected in any crisis disease of the thyroid. Once it is eliminated, often, function returns to normal.

The ovaries are critical organs that are directly integrated with rest of the endocrine system. Yet, physicians feel little hesitation of removing them. Can a man imagine what it would be like to have the testicles cut off? Ovaries are their equals. For any disease process removing the testicles should be the absolute last resort. Yet, the surgeon is often cavalier taking them out. out the ovaries. This is despite the fact that this devastates a female's health, including that of the thyroid gland. It was Larson who claimed that there is no greater harm done to the female body than the inappropriate removal of these organs. He makes it clear that even in the event of known pathology every effort should be made only to remove the diseased tissue. Any possible part of the ovary which might be healthy, he says, must be salvaged.

When a woman's ovaries are removed, it is highly traumatic. This is an essential organ, which is involved in operations far more complex than sexual activity alone. The ovaries support a woman's entire hormone system. They are needed to help keep this system in a finely tuned balance. Helping to maintain metabolism throughout the body, especially in the adrenal and thyroid glands, when these organs are removed, the entire endocrine system is placed into disarray. Great strain is usually placed on the thyroid gland, and it usually fails.

When even a single ovary is removed, a woman's femininity is distorted. Critical functions or aspects, including the inclination for lovemaking, natural feminine vitality, body conformation, healthy mood/mental state, and menstruation, cease or are disrupted. The natural spark, so prominent in vital women, escapes, never to again return. The same consequence results in men whose prostate glands are removed or who lose testes. They, too, lack that vital essence, which makes a man so sensual. Yet, through the intake of natural hormones and the proper nutritional supplements some of this essence can be resurrected. Part of this can be accomplished by boosting sister glands, such as thyroid and adrenals, which compensate for this loss. When the ovaries fail or when they are weak, there are certain physical signs. One of these involves fat distribution. An ovarian fat pad develops on the lateral hip. When this is seen, it is a sign that the woman is an ovarian type.

The age factor

Sluggish thyroid function is a consequence of aging. Virtually everyone suffers a decline in the powers of this gland with time. As described by Mohandas and Gupta in their article *Managing Thyroid Dysfunction in the Elderly* (May 2003) there are certain specific symptoms which are revealing. These include slowing of mental function (poor concentration), poor memory, high cholesterol, intolerance to cold, dryness of the skin, exhaustion, muscular weakness, constipation, poor concentration, and hoarseness. Even deafness can indicate hypothyroidism.

In rare instances the elderly could develop excessive thyroid function, that is hyperthyroidism. This is manifested by rapid heartbeat, weight loss, fatigue, nervousness, agitation, tremors, excessive urination, intolerance to heat, and excessive sweating. This most commonly occurs in younger people aged 20 through 45. Usually, elderly people suffer with hypothyroidism. This may be manifested by a modest amount of symptoms: mere tiredness and poor circulation, perhaps with muscular weakness and a degree of sluggish mentation. This why in the elderly the diagnosis of sluggish thyroid syndrome is frequently missed.

Chapter Three

Diet and Nutrition

Diet profoundly influences thyroid function. This gland, while damaged by stress, is even more greatly disrupted by a toxic diet. Also, it is readily damaged by specific deficiencies, notably a lack of iodine, amino acids, riboflavin, thiamine, niacin, magnesium, and zinc. Incredibly, a simple deficiency of iodine and amino acids causes extensive damage of this gland. If the deficiency is prolonged or extreme, it may undergo atrophy, that is permanent cell death. A deficiency in B vitamins can also result in similar consequences.

In the early 1900s before the role of nutritional deficiency in this organ was firmly established millions of people all over the world suffered from severe thyroid disease. This was in the form of goiter. This is a type of cellular degeneration. The cells over-grow–or hypertrophy– destroying the infrastructure of the gland. It is all preventable, as well as reversible, strictly through improved nutrition. Iodine is the main deficiency, but, again, there are a wide range of nutrients lacking. Goiter is essentially a gross nutritional deficiency, complicated by overall glandular imbalances. That's why most efficient treatment for goiter involves treating the entire endocrine system.

There is another major factor besides deficiency. This is anti-thyroid substances. Incredibly, in nature there are a number of substances, which block iodine absorption. What's more, these substances appear to directly interfere with the action of thyroid hormones. Known as goitrogens, they are found exclusively in vegetation, particularly raw vegetation.

Common vegetables are the major sources of goitrogens. These include primarily vegetables from the mustard family, notably turnips and radishes as well as the cruciferous vegetables, that is Brussels sprouts, cabbage, broccoli, kohlrabi, and cauliflower. Raw carrots and, therefore, carrot juice also contain these compounds. In a severely thyroid-deficient individual the regular consumption of such vegetables may aggravate the condition. In some cases, incredibly, overeating such vegetables may even cause the disorder. In the early 1900s this was well recognized, McCarrison deeming it "cabbage goiter."

Other sources of goitrogens include raw flaxseed (and, therefore, raw flaxseed oil), raw peanuts, raw almonds, raw walnuts, and raw strawberries. Soy, raw or cooked, is also a major perpetrator. In particular, soy concentrates, such as soy protein, curd, and milk, vigorously block thyroid function. This is particularly true for unfermented sources, which retain the full strength of the toxins.

Now that soy is genetically engineered its toxicity is greatly increased. No one should eat commercial soy products. This is particularly true of people with thyroid disorders, who should avoid all these soy foods and various derivatives like the plague. Thyroid types must be particularly careful about soy or its derivatives.

Goitrogens are metabolic inhibitors. Such substances are cyanogenic glycosides, which are a biological form of cyanide. Any chemist knows that cyanide is a metabolic poison. This is why such substances can be so dangerous to the thyroid gland, since it has the highest metabolic rate in the body and is, therefore, highly sensitive to these poisons.

Consider a person living in central or eastern Europe, eating little or no fish and using little if any salt. Then, such a person eats large amounts of traditional foods. These foods include raw cabbage, sauerkraut, Brussels sprouts, raw carrots, cauliflower, radishes, and turnips. As a result, the person becomes lethargic and depressed, even hostile. The throat and neck swell. Here, it is still known as cabbage goiter. Cabbage and similar cruciferous vegetables are consumed in large amounts in central and eastern Europe. No wonder sluggish thyroid syndrome is a plague in this region.

The general rule is avoidance of all processed foods. The thyroid gland was not made to deal with these. Plus, these foods and beverage are depleted in the necessary mineral salts, naturally occurring sodium, chloride, iodine, magnesium, zinc, and copper, upon which the organ thrives. People with thyroid disorders must read labels carefully.

A high-grain diet is also destructive to the thyroid. This again has to do with tissue salt-bearing foods. Grains contain virtually none of these salts. What's more, they are devoid of iodine, whereas meats, fish, milk, cheese, and eggs, all of which are salt bearing, are ◆relatively rich. This is particularly true of such animal foods derived from lands high in iodine such as the meat from cattle grazing in Florida, North and South Carolina, Virginia, New Jersey, New York, Ireland/England, and similar iodine-rich regions. Regardless, animal foods are far denser in this substance than vegetation, the exception being sea vegetables.

The strict exclusion of animal foods ultimately leads to thyroid decay, that is unless the diet is regularly supplemented with sea vegetation and/or thyroid glandulars. People say meat is bad but not from an endocrinological point of view. Its tissue salts fuel the endocrine system in ways that no vegetable can do so. There is also carnitine in animal foods, which is needed for fuel generation in the thyroid. Thus, the ideal nutritional support for this organ would include, perhaps, a combination of iodine-rich vegetation, such as low-pollution kelp/seaweed, and animal sources such as fresh beef, lamb, organ meat, eggs, fatty fish, and whole milk. Regarding eggs, their content of iodine is directly related to the feed. If it is lacking, the eggs will not be a good source.

Elimination of animal-source foods leads to a corresponding deficiency of food salts, including iodine and chloride. There is also a reduction in the intake of hormones, which are concentrated mainly in animal flesh. This includes muscle meat. If suffering from a thyroid problem, don't think of meat as a poison or 'dead' food, as is commonly written. Consider it as a means to achieve the necessary nutrition for optimal endocrine function.

So, what would be an ideal thyroid-support diet. It would contain the following foods and beverages:

- grass-fed meat
- truly free-range poultry
- grass-fed organ meats
- fatty fish and seafood
- grass-fed whole milk products
- range-free and organic eggs
- fresh, organic greens and wild greens
- green and red sweet peppers, possibly yellow versions
- fresh fruit in season
- brown and wild rice
- sweet potatoes (ideally raw in salads)
- Jerusalem and regular artichokes

- eggplant and tomatoes
- avocadoes and olives
- brans of cereal grains (as a source of soluble fiber and B vitamins)
- nuts and seeds

Notice that food high in starch, like whole wheat, white flour, corn, potatoes, and rye, are off the list or at least their consumption is limited. So is the intake of pork, which is, regardless, difficult to digest. As well, the consumption of nitrated meats is banned, as this food leads to a serious increased risk of cancer and heart disease.

One key is grass-fed meat consumption. So is the intake, if possible, of grass-fed organ meat. Quality poultry with the skin on is another supreme food. These meat sources will provide thyroid hormones and various hormone precursors lodged in the flesh, which cannot be procured in vegetation. The exception is kelp, which is a dense source of such precursors as well as iodine. For vegans it is essential to add high-quality kelp sources to the thyroid treatment profile. Yet, as a rule, a purely vegetable diet poses extreme challenges for nourishing this gland. Long-term veganism may cause a complete shutdown of this system, leading to a form of hypothyroidism complicated by extreme alkalosis. This may precipitate fungal infection. Vegans who suffer health problems should be sure to take oil of wild oregano and a wild oregano herbal mix with Rhus coriaria, as a means to neutralize this.

As many as one in four Americans suffer from reduced thyroid function. Low body temperature is perhaps the most common consequence of impaired thyroid function. The individual who wears extra layers of clothes, wears socks to bed, or who has "ice cold hands" is typically thyroid deficient. This lowered body core temperature affects several critical functions, including digestive enzyme synthesis, stomach acid production, fuel combustion, fat and protein synthesis, white blood cell synthesis/activity, and blood flow. The thyroid gland is also a critical player in the synthesis and activity of sex hormones, so, usually, in hypofunction the blood levels of these hormones are low.

In this syndrome immunity is compromised. This is a consequence of the reduced enzyme activity. It is also because of the reduction in body temperature. The immune system operates best at the normal temperature of 98.6 degrees Fahrenheit or higher. When the body is constantly in a low temperature, immune activity is sluggish. This increases the vulnerability for opportunistic infections, particularly fungal infections. In fact, one of the cardinal features of a sluggish thyroid is persistent fungal infections of the skin, scalp, and nails. Also, persistent psoriasis and/or eczema is often a signal of sluggish thyroid function.

As well, in hypothyroidism fungus readily populates the deeper tissues, including the internal organs, blood, and bone marrow. The low body core temperature greatly increases the risks for deep-seated fungal infections; the immune system simply doesn't have the capacity to clear these organisms. In hypothyroidism even the white blood cells prove to be incompetent. This creates the environment that allows these pathogens to thrive. Actually, the majority of people with toenail fungus are the thyroid type. The same is true with those suffering from persistent cases of athlete's foot.

Psoriasis and eczema are related to germ overgrowth. One reason for this is low oxygen levels in the tissues, which is typical of depressed thyroid function. This leads to the overgrowth of pathogens, such as fungi, strep, and staph, therefore causing the skin lesions.

Fat metabolism

There are real problems in fat metabolism with this insufficiency. Often, there are excessive fats and lipids in the blood, which can pose a serious problem with circulation. In the extreme the poorly metabolized fats and lipids can form clots, leading to acute or chronic clots in the legs and lungs. Even more dangerous is accumulation in the coronary arteries, leading to heart attack or other clots sent the brain, causing strokes. Regardless, a high cholesterol and/or triglyceride are common signs of a thyroid disorder. So is fatty liver.

Much of this excessive accumulations is related not to fat intake, such as the eating of eggs and meat, but, rather, the consumption of starch. Pure carbohydrate, with thyroid dysfunction it cannot be burned efficiently, and so it is turned into fatty acids and cholesterol. This is done in the liver and, often, excesses are lodged in that organ, and it is weighed down with fatty accumulations. It all has to be burned out by boosting the metabolic rate to normal.

Nutrients needed by the thyroid

Much of it has already been discussed. Yet, there is value in summarizing the nutrients required by this metabolically active gland. Incredibly, it amounts to the majority of the key nutrients known. The most obvious one is iodine, which the thyroid specifically concentrates. Of the normal mass of this gland is found the iodinated protein, thyroglobulin. This is the basis for the formation of the active compound, T3, which as is indicated contains three iodine molecules. The iodine is so crucial that, without it, active thyroid hormone cannot be formed. The gland also needs the amino acid tyrosine, the base molecule for the hormone's formation.

Iodine can be found in seafood, grass-fed meat, eggs, and poultry. Kelp is the richest natural source. Too much of this substance, though, can pose a problem, causing toxicity of this gland and even leading the dangerous states of Hashimoto's disease and hyperthyroidism.

Other key nutrients include a variety of minerals, especially iron, zinc, and selenium. Vitamins A and D are much needed, as is the B complex, especially niacin and thiamine. The essential fatty acids and vitamin C round the list. In particular, a lack of vitamin A causes the gland to degenerate, as does a deficiency in zinc. The latter is required as well for the conversion of T4 into the more active form, T3.

Substances that work against the thyroid, depleting its nutrients, include common bad habit materials such as alcohol, tobacco, and refined sugar. Other anti-thyroid elements include herbicides, pesticides, certain antibiotics, chlorine, perchlorate, bisphenols, dioxins, PCBs, and fluoride. In addition, the heavy metals cadmium, lead, aluminum, and mercury are highly poisonous to this gland. If any of these are overloaded in the body, they should be flushed out. Ideal natural medicines for this include the Intestimax and PlumClenz.

Chapter Four

Weathering the Storm

When it comes to temperature, thyroid types do have their preferences. They enjoy warm or moderate weather. In contrast, they complain bitterly about the cold or even a chilly wind. Wet, cool weather isn't much better. When exposed, as well, it may take them an inordinate amount of time to warm up. With exposure to cold the body is normally driven into action with a sudden increase in thyroid hormone synthesis. Not so with those with weakened thyroids, the system simply cannot respond. From the pituitary TSH is supposed to pour out under the cold stress to compensate. Yet, it doesn't, and so the thyroid can't raise the core temperature. Thus, when exposed to the cold, the hypothyroid person often has the opposite effect, becoming colder and more intolerant with every cold stressor. This is why in the winter months such a one often adds layers of extra clothes, the only effective compensation.

Frequently, the hypothyroid person will say, "Is it cold in here?" adding, "I am cold. Can anyone turn up the heat?" With this propensity it is difficult for them to operate in chilly weather. After all, they are grossly deficient. The thyroid gland is the body's thermoregulation mechanism. One of its major jobs is to create body heat, largely from the combustion of calories and oxygen. When exposed, its job is to react efficiently, so that the cold is not so bothersome. Basically, it acts to increase metabolic actions to warm a person up—or it is supposed to. Yet, since it is sluggish the chilly weather amounts to just one more stress upon the gland. As a result, the lowered temperature can cause a person to suffer an exacerbation, to actually be irritable, depressed, and fatigued, even agitated, even during the winter to gain weight.

Clearly, with the frigidness the thyroid is forced to work harder, much more so than it is capable. In fact, the body uses up the hormone, where the T4 and T3 levels typically drop, a disaster for the hypothyroid case. To help avoid this it is necessary to "dress-up" for the winter and avoid unnecessary stressful exposures, while also increasing the intake of the thyroid-supporting supplements mentioned in this book.

Top supplements for warming up include a complex of kelp plus the amino acid. Yet another is the Body Shape Code thyroid supplement made with New Zealand glandulars. Yet another is the microcirculation-enhancing sour grape powder. Adding high-quality sea salt to the diet is also advised. All these will aid the body in fighting back against the cold intolerance. It is important to watch the symptoms to be sure they improve. Low body core temperature increases the risks for cardiovascular conditions and also fungal infection. The risk for cancer is considerably higher, as low body core temperature is a carcinogenic state. Of note, cancer is impaired by heat, plus the normal heat index helps motivate the natural production in the bone marrow of white blood cells.

There is the issue of both a drop in body core temperature and the slowing of metabolism. There are the main symptoms of both feeling cold constantly and being intolerant to it when exposed. These symptoms must be evaluated to see how effective the therapy is. It is critical to raise the metabolism and, therefore, the core temperature. This can also be followed with the underarm temperature test. When it reaches around 97.6 or more, that is a sign of strong, improved metabolism.

The slowdown is complete

With inadequate thyroid hormones or their impaired function there are many aspects of the body which go into a depressed mode. The body goes into a virtual hibernation mode. The combustion of food is tremendously slowed. A person can't burn the carbohydrates, digest properly the food, motivate adequately the immune system, fight reasonably against the cold, think sharply and clearly, and maintain a heart that pumps strongly. What more could go wrong in this slow-down? Actually, there is more. The lungs become dysfunctional, and the metabolic activity the pancreas and liver dramatically decline.

The skin and muscle may systematically degenerate; cellularly, the muscles simply break down, where they cannot contract strongly—and this may be the mechanism in the heart itself. In the brain the ability of this organ to utilize oxygen and other nutrients declines dramatically, especially if myxedematous fluids infiltrate it. In the throat and bronchial tree there is a collapse of normal mucous formation; great dryness may result. Thus, a person can often hardly swallow or breathe. The muscle activity of the esophagus may decline, with the contractile fibers degenerating. This can be serious; the person can choke to death. This happened to Mama Cass of the Mamas & Papas, who was clearly a thyroid type. Had she been diagnosed and treated adequately, she wouldn't have choked to death on that meat.

The intestines, too, can suffer a horrific slow-down. There is the issue of peristalsis, as in the esophagus, all the way down. What of the production of hydrochloric acid and digestive enzymes? All this is reduced or upended. Thyroid hormone is needed for enzyme activity, which are dependent upon body temperature. If the core temperature is reduced, enzyme function plummets. The production of mucous also falters, so needed for the intestinal lining health. Constipation ultimately strikes, and the hypothyroid person often observes that food "just sits" and doesn't efficiently digest.

Chapter Five

Thyroid Self-Test

To determine thyroid status the following test is provided. Based upon careful research and assessment this test can be used as a thyroid health guidance system. Use such tests, plus the diagrams and signs listed in this book, to determine your status. Blood tests may also be taken. For making an assessment the combination of the written tests plus blood tests is a good idea. However, for simplicity most people can determine their status through the information found in this book. A score in the moderate category or greater indicates that the person is primarily a thyroid type. A similar test can be found on www.ebodytype.com. There, an individual's results will be recorded by membership for repeating the results. This is a thorough test, more so than any blood tests can achieve. If there is any degree of hypothyroidism, it will be uncovered through this self-test. The system encourages follow-up, necessary to evaluate the effectiveness of therapy. Note: it is helpful to take this test while before a mirror:

Thyroid type self-test:

Which of these apply to you (each response worth one point, unless otherwise indicated)?

•fatigue or tiredness (2)

- tired in the morning and energetic at night (3 points)
- dry or coarse hair,
- hair is brittle and snaps off
- alopecia
- bore of the hair is thick
- slow or slurred speech (2 points)
- little-to-no desire to eat (2)
- bloating and indigestion after eating (stomach blows up)
- mouth is excessively dry even if drinking water•poor muscular tone (flabbiness)
- anemia
- white count is too low
  —moderately (2)
  —severely (3)
- puffiness of the face
- swelling or puffiness about the eyes and/or on eyelids (2)
- swelling/puffiness of hands and/or ankles (2 points)
- cold hands and feet (2 points)
- failure to thrive in youth or adolescence (3)
- hair loss from the outer third of the eyebrows (3 points)
- hair loss from scalp
  —male, who is becoming bald and losing hair from the front back (3)
  —woman, whose hair is thinning
  moderately (3)
  severely (4)
- short-term memory loss (2 points)
- white spots on the fingernails
- chronic weight problems
- easily constipated (3 points)

THE HEALTH BENEFITS OF THYROID METABO... 31

- eat and the food sits like a rock, doesn't digest (2)
- undigested food in the stool
- diagnosed with low or no stomach acid, that is hypochlorhydria or achlorhydria (2)
- PMS
- excessive periods (menorrhagia) (2)
- lack of periods (amenorrhea)
- uterine fibroids
  — moderate (2)
  — severe (3)
- infertility
- chronic headaches, especially after age 40 (2 points)
  — headaches are daily or nearly that, low-grade (3)
- brittle nails or nails which grow slowly)
- mental sluggishness and/or confusion
- low motivation
- heart palpitations
- drink fluoridated and/or chlorinated water or
- use fluoridated toothpastes and/or rinses
- index finger is shorter than the ring finger on both hands
  — obviously shorter on both hands (4)
  — not so obvious but shorter (3)
- joint stiffness
- require prolonged periods to get "warmed up" after exposure to cold (2 points)
- lack of sexual desire
- apathy
- vulnerable to infections, especially by yeast
- enlarged facial pores
- poor hand-to-eye coordination

- hoarseness or coarse voice not related to smoking (3 points)
- inability to translate thoughts into action (2 points)
- become depressed in the winter
- don't feel like getting up in the morning and often shut the alarm off repeatedly (3 points)
- history of ovarian cysts
  —moderate (2)
  —severe (3)
- lived in the Great Lakes region for over ten years—Illinois, Wisconsin, Indiana, Michigan, Ohio or in Canada, Manitoba, Saskatchewan, and Ontario (2 points)
- high cholesterol level (2 points)
- cholesterol deposits on face and elsewhere (xanthomas)
- high triglycerides
- rarely or never eat ocean fish and/or seafood (2)
- rarely or never consume sea vegetables or kelp (3)
- on a strict low-salt diet
- rarely or never consume red meat
- have multiple silver-mercury fillings
  —up to four (2)
  —five or more (3)
- toenail or fingernail fungal infections
- skin fungal infections, including psoriasis or eczema
- head is square or rectangular in shape (2 points
- sleep until noon (3 points)
- lack of moons (light colored semicircles) on the index, middle, and ring fingers (2 points)
- history of heart disease, mitral valve prolapse, and/or congestive heart failure (3)
- atrial fibrillation

THE HEALTH BENEFITS OF THYROID METABO... 33

—occasional (2)

—persistent (3)

- heart rate is excessively slow (below 62 without exercise) (2)
- high blood pressure

—moderate (2)

—severe (3)

- thick multiple vertical ridges on the nails
- deep horizontal ridges on the nails
- large, bulbous, thick tongue (floppy tongue)
- sluggish digestion
- poor circulation
- furrows on the brow
- corners of the eyes droop downwards
- top lip is excessively thin
- development of crows feet about the eyes
- outer corners of the mouth droop downwards
- love handles on the back
- follicular hyperkeratosis (enlarged pores or bumps on back of upper arms)
- �apple-shaped body, that is an upside-down apple 3 points)
- gain weight mainly on front of abdomen, usually no more than 20 pounds (3 points)
- chronic heartburn/indigestion
- taking Paxil, Zoloft, Prozac, or other antidepressants on a regular basis
- history of pernicious anemia
- dry, coarse skin
- muscle cramps
- decreased memory, especially short-term
- numbness and tingling

- impaired hearing
- decreased sweating
- chronic yeast infections
—moderate (2)
—severe (3)
- coarseness and hoarseness of the voice, including loss in women of naturally sweet tone (3)
  - hand and finger swelling, also of the face, legs, and arm
  - Do you drink alcohol on a daily or weekly basis?
—moderately (2)
—to the extreme (3)
- Do you smoke tobacco on a daily basis?
—not much, like five or less cigarettes (2)
—moderately (3)
—extremely (4)
- Do you regularly consume chlorinated water without filtering it?
- Do you use chlorine or bleach commonly in your cleaning?
- Do you rely on coffee to 'wake up' in the morning? 2
- Drink excessive amounts of coffee or other caffeinated drinks:
—one to three drinks daily 1
—four to six drinks daily 2
—more than six drinks daily 3
- Do you suffer from fatty liver? (2)
- Do you suffer from diabetes type 2?
—mild case (pre- or early-diabetes)
—moderate case (3)
—severe case (4)
- elevated glycosylated hemoglobin (2)
  - Have you received radiation treatments to the head, neck, and/or chest? (3)

- Have you received chest X-rays—three to five (2)
- —six to 10 (3)
- —more than 10 (4)
- Have you had your thyroid removed?

partially (3)

totally (5)

- Have you taken radioactive iodine as a thyroid medical treatment? (4)
- Have you had dental CT-Scans?

a few (2)

more than four (3)

- Have you had whole-body CT-Scans?

one to two 3

two to four 4

more than four (5)

- Have you been pregnant?

one to three times (2)

four to five times (3)

more than five times (4)

Your score_____

One to 6 points, Likely thyroid insufficiency: While this is not definitive evidence, still, an early thyroid insufficiency is likely. Regardless, it is a good idea to increase the consumption of foods rich in hormonal agents such as grass-fed red meat, organic poultry with the skin on, whole milk foods, organic eggs, and wild seafood. Ashwagandha extract and royal jelly are ideal supportive supplements as is kelp.

7 to 13 points, mild thyroid insufficiency: At this level supplementation is advised. Take the Body Shape Diet/Code thyroid-support supplement, two capsules daily. As well, increase the consumption of foods rich in hormonal agents such as grass-fed red meat, organic poultry with the skin on, whole milk foods, organic eggs, and wild seafood. Avoid all refined food, especially sugar and starch, while also avoiding alcohol and caffeine.

14 to 23 points, moderate thyroid insufficiency: Take the Body Shape Diet/Code thyroid-support supplement, two capsules twice daily. Also, consume the ashwagandha concentrate capsules with organic royal jelly, two caps twice daily. As well, increase the consumption of foods rich in hormonal agents such as grass-fed red meat, organic poultry with the skin on, whole milk foods, organic eggs, and wild seafood. Avoid all refined food, especially sugar and starch, while also avoiding alcohol and caffeine. Take the key nutrients needed for healthy thyroid function in a whole food form. Take a B Complex, ADK, and a natural whole food Vitamin C. Also, consume Zinc daily.

24 to 32 points, severe thyroid insufficiency: Take the Body Shape Diet/Code thyroid-support supplement, three capsules daily twice daily. Also, consume the ashwagandha concentrate capsules with organic royal jelly, three caps twice daily. As well, increase the consumption of foods rich in hormonal agents such as grass-fed red meat, organic poultry with the skin on, whole milk foods, organic eggs, and wild seafood. Avoid all refined food, especially sugar and starch, while also avoiding alcohol and caffeine. Take a B Complex, ADK, and a natural whole food Vitamin C. Also, consume Zinc daily. Take also the oil of wild oregano as well as the juice-essence, five drops twice daily of the oil and two T. of the juice.

33 to 39 points, extreme thyroid insufficiency: Take the Body Shape Diet or Body Shape Code thyroid-support supplement, four or more capsules twice daily. Also, consume an ashwagandha concentrate as well as pure royal jelly, 2 times daily. In females if the ovaries are sluggish, add a blend of kelp with Mediterranean oregano, black seed and sumac – 2X per day. As well, increase the consumption of foods rich in hormonal agents such as grass-fed red meat, organic poultry with the skin on, whole milk foods, organic eggs, and wild seafood. Avoid all refined food, especially sugar and starch, while also avoiding alcohol and caffeine. This is a serious level of deficiency and may require medication. Ideally, the naturalistic approach will suffice. Have your doctor follow your case with the appropriate blood tests to be sure there is steady improvement. Take a natural whole food B Complex. Also, consume natural pure zinc, 2 T. daily. Fungal overload may be complicating the hypothyroid state. Take also the oil of wild oregano as well as the juice-essence, five drops twice daily of the oil and two T. of the juice twice daily. The juice is particularly valuable for eliminating thyroid nodules as well as goiter.

40 and above, profoundly extreme thyroid insufficiency: Take the Body Shape Diet thyroid-support supplement, four or more capsules twice daily. Also, consume an ashwagandha concentrate as well as pure royal jelly, 2 times daily. In females if the ovaries are sluggish, add a blend of kelp with Mediterranean oregano, black seed and sumac – 3X per day. As well, increase the consumption of foods rich in hormonal agents such as grass-fed red meat, organic poultry with the skin on, whole milk foods, organic eggs, and wild seafood. Avoid all refined food, especially sugar and starch, while also avoiding alcohol and caffeine. This is a serious level of deficiency and may require medication. Ideally, the naturalistic approach will suffice. Have your doctor follow your case with the appropriate blood tests to be sure there is steady improvement. Take a natural whole food B Complex. Also, consume natural pure zinc, three T. daily. Fungal overload may be complicating the hypothyroid state. Take also the oil of wild oregano as well as the juice-essence, five drops twice daily of the oil and two T. of the juice twice daily. The juice is particularly valuable for eliminating thyroid nodules as well as goiter.

Note: chlorine and fluoride are highly poisonous to this gland and block the uptake of the critically needed iodine, even displacing the molecule from active positions on the hormone.

While this testing is through it may seem complicated to some people. As a rule, there is a general assessment that is more simplistic. People with extreme thyroid disorders develop a certain look. They appear puffy or swollen. Their faces droop downward. More sluggish than others their minds don't seem to work right—not as fast and alert as others. Complaining, they have constant digestive problems. Sluggish thyroid syndrome cases suffer from an obvious thickness, even if not obese. This thickness is of the extremities, face, and torso. The tissue can be pressed on and manipulated, but it does not feel to be blubber. It can only be imagined what is happening internally. Yet, they are the first ones to develop heart disease, cancer, arthritis, and diabetes. Reading this may aid in making a quick assessment of the case.

There is another curious self-test that may be applied. This is evidence for oxygen deficiency. The metabolism of this gas within the tissues is under thyroid control. Let us see what the score in oxygen-handling capacity is, though some of these questions are repetition of the major test:

- complete lack of moons on index, ring, and middle fingers: 5
- partial lack of moons on index, ring, and middle fingers (3)
- too much reddish color more than the normal light pink in nail beds (2)
- face is excessively reddish, particularly the cheeks
- rosacea

—moderate (2)

—severe (3)
- blood vessel engorgement on the upper checks, where the tiny capillaries can be seen.

—mild (2)

—moderate (3)

—severe (4)
- injection of blood vessels in whites of eyes
- can't get a deep breath (2)
- impaired mental function, including taking excessively long time to put thoughts together.
- difficult time arising from sleep (2)
- difficult time falling to sleep (2)
- chronic headaches

—moderate (2)

—severe and/or daily (3)
- no desire for exercise (2)
- poor recovery from exercise and/or easily get out of breath
- muscles have no tone despite exercise (flabby)
- develop internal cancers easily (2)
- would like to do work and activity but feel like it is impossible, ¬¬become overwhelmed (2)
- continuously feel sleepy despite sleeping sufficiently
- eyes feel heavy
- heart feels heavy, with action being slow or weak (2)
- constantly depressed despite medication

Any score of four or more is a sign of sluggish thyroid-induced oxygen deficiency. A score of five to 10 indicates a significant lack of this gas; it may well be consumed, breathed in, but it is not being metabolized. At the level of 11 to 18 this is a sign of severe oxygen deficit and indicates an incompetence of thyroid function. Anyone who scores above 18 is monumentally severely deficient in this gas, metabolically.

Think about it. The body is doing all it can to gain oxygenation. There is even the enlargement of blood vessels on the corneas of the eyes and on the cheeks. Incredibly, this is to capture this gas from the air about the body, all largely because it is being so inefficiently used in the tissues. All these signs and symptoms should improve as thyroid function is restored. Keep track of them; score them from one to five, the latter being the worst. Then, the results should be re-evaluated after therapy is applied. As thyroid hormone controls all oxygenation gaining more of it will work towards correcting this. This is a major effort, combining sound diet and exercise with nutritional supplementation. Suddenly, the body will be vitalized to use the oxygen it receives. The correct selection of food plus supplements and sound exercise will all make the difference in this correction. Take pictures, too, so there can be definitive before-and-after data.

Chapter Six

Conclusion

It is a serious issue to have significant thyroid dysfunction. The test, combined with underarm temperature results, gives an accurate assessment of thyroid status. If dysfunctional, there is no means for the body to operate efficiently. Without a functioning gland the body will not be able to do the most basic tasks, like breaking down proteins. It cannot process and metabolism carbohydrates and sugar. Even vitamins are poorly metabolism. Because of the food metabolic instability this explains the potential for uncontrollable weight gain. Its control-powers are truly immense. If the body is in disarray, the thyroid is involved. Yet, how did the individual score? Where all the systems in some level of dysfunction? How was the breathing, heart function, hair and skin health, circulatory capacity, lymph function, muscle strength or lack thereof, menstrual cycle, cholesterol levels, body temperature, and brain function—all represent tell-tale signs, because they are all under thyroid control.

Yet, as mentioned, the brain itself is heavily involved in hormonal function. Specifically, it is the hypothalamus and pituitary that modulate the key thyroid hormone levels: T3 and T4. If the system works adequately, it is all kept under a tight control. So, in hypothyroidism a serious metabolic disruption has occurred, since this is in violation of all that the body seeks to do. Then, again, to suffer with depression, insomnia, exhaustion, poor concentration, dry skin/hair/membranes, and muscle or joint pain is a major issue. This is especially true since these are consequences of failed glandular function—plus, this is often brought on by stress but also nutritional deficiency.

It is astounding that all this could be related to a single organ system. Yet, there is hope in this fact. A concentrated program aimed at this functionality could result in a broad scope of improvement. A person could become well just be placing, once and for all, the thyroid in a strong balance. This could prove life changing. As well, it could be the factor behind preventing the onset of debilitating illnesses and also premature death.

It is clearly the case. A person goes to the doctor with heart rhythm disturbances, diagnosed as atrial fibrillation. Medication is prescribed, but if this fails, a surgical procedure is applied, an ablation, which amounts to permanently destroying cardiac nerves, Then, an artifice is added, a pacemaker, which is implanted. Yet, this is all a false approach. The man, obese on the front, tired, and suffering overall poor circulation plus insomnia—hypothyroidism was the cause. If this was treated appropriately, the atrial fibrillation would have disappeared, the heart rate regulated by the normalized thyroid function. It was all a waste plus a significant danger to his system. No one followed the physiology.

So, what happened in this case? With impaired thyroid capacity the heart becomes weak. T3 is required for its ability to pump and also for cardiac muscular tone. As a result, the muscle becomes flaccid and even enlarged. With this weak stroke or pumping it reacts by fibrillating, because this is a danger—people feel the aberrant sensation and also there is a high risk of clot formation and, therefore, strokes—physicians react. This is the basis of the draconian procedures.

A woman suffers from uterine enlargement plus growths, that is fibroids. Over 50 and after having several children, she begins bleeding excessively, leading to anemia. With failure of medication doctor act and cut out her uterus, possibly ovaries. No one paid attention to the fact that she was moderately obese, extremely sensitive to cold, tired, is a fairly strict vegetarian, and was losing her hair. The cause of the uterine growths was sluggish thyroid syndrome. If this was aggressively addressed, the bleeding could have been halted and the fibroids likely would recede.

An early adolescent has failure to thrive. Additionally, there is poor dental formation as well as delayed sexual maturation. No one knows what to do; doctors are befuddled, and the parents deeply concerned. They attempt numerous medications and altering the diet to no avail. He is shorter than his age average, and students are making fun of him. Yet, he is chubby, always tired, sleeps to noon unless aroused, and his grades are suffering. He also has massive white spots on his nails. He, too, has hypothyroidism, and the white spots are tell-tale. This gland is dependent upon zinc for thyroid hormone synthesis. They reveal that the child is gluten intolerant, which leads to zinc malabsorption by causing the destruction of the intestinal villi. Plus, in some individual this grain protein is directly poisonous to the gland itself. Correction of the diet to gluten-free, the giving of a whole food zinc supplement, and the treatment of the thyroid disorder could well result in restitution of normal growth.

A 40-year-old woman suffers from extreme degrees of exhaustion. This seems to be related to her veganism, which she adopted over a decade ago. Anything animal she won't touch. In addition, she is severely sensitive to cold. Also suffering from sluggishness, she is having difficulty with her mental function, having a hard time with her thoughts and forming sentences.

Clinching the diagnosis: hand signs

No doubt, the tests aid greatly in this assessment. "Am I truly a thyroid type?" Everyone must know. Yet, the underarm temperature testing is also of great value. However, there is a simple way to be relatively sure. This is the body shape and also the finger length. This is true of both the thyroid type and its subsidiary, the thyroid-adrenal type.

To determine this place the hands, fingers together, on a surface. Using the dominant eye attempt to evaluate the finger-length. If the first finger is shorter than the ring finger (4th digit) on both hands, obviously so, this is the classical thyroid type. If the first finger is just shorter on both hands, it is still thyroid but is closer to a thyroid-adrenal type. If the finger on the dominant hand is shorter but the one on the other hand is actually the same length or longer, this is a thyroid-adrenal type (see Figures 2).

If the shape of the body is similar to an upside-down apple, this is additional hard proof of the thyroid type. This is especially true if there is no obvious grith in the buttocks and if the sides of the thighs are relatively flat. If it is more like a big, long watermelon, this more likely indicates a thyroid-adrenal representation (see Figure 3).

When the hands of this type are viewed, typically, the index fingers are one of four representations, although the one already mentioned is the most common:

- they are just short compared to the ring finger
- one is shorter, and the other is longer or the same length
- they are both the same length as the index fingers

Regardless, a person combines this definitive data to the other information found here and comes to the appropriate conclusion. These

THE HEALTH BENEFITS OF THYROID METABO...

are astounding findings of great value for endocrine health, the first time ever been published. Now, it is possible to determine the thyroid status without undergoing potentially expensive and invasive tests.

There are a few other characteristics of this type. Instead of coarse hair, as seen in a pure thyroid, it is medium-coarse. There may be the holding of some weight in the abdomen, but not as much as the true thyroid type. In addition, they may only be somewhat tired in the morning and less sensitive to cold temperature. Plus, the underarm temperature tends to be higher, almost never as low as 95 to 96 degrees; usually, but not always, above 97. If it is in the lower digits, then that means the thyroid component is significant. The rule is for determining this type is that the dominant hand has the short index finger, while with the other one it is either longer, just shorter, or the same length.

Thyroid-adrenal type: the approach

The endocrine glands work as a team. If the thyroid is weakened, then the adrenals will be disturbed as a result. It is a compensatory mechanism. In order to achieve optimal health both must be treated. Often, as well, the gonads are incapacitated. These, too, must be put into balance to achieve optimal results.

The approach to the thyroid-adrenal type is slightly different than for the pure thyroid case. There must be an effort to also balance adrenal function. There is a body shape code adrenal formula which can be added to the thyroid formula. Take at least two capsules of each twice daily. For both thyroid and adrenal support ashwagandha concentrate should be consumed, that is the 10:1 extract It is also advisable to increase salt consumption; the Triple Salt Caps would be ideal, about two capsules twice daily. A low salt diet is a catastrophe in the event of an adrenal component. The diet is essentially the same as the thyroid type, although the combination person can generally handle more carbohydrate than the pure thyroid type. This is especially true if the person tends not to put on weight on the abdomen.

The adrenal glands control circulation. This is through maintaining blood volume. In order to do so they conserve salt. In fact, if there is a craving for salt, this is one of the major signs of the adrenal component. Blood sugar regulation is also under their management. This is a major issue, and if the adrenals are weak, there will be a variety of related symptoms. These symptoms include fatigue, which can be extreme, headache, nervousness, anxiety, depression, apprehensions, obsessiveness, insomnia, poor concentration, light headedness, anger/agitation fits, and fainting spells or nearly fainting spells. In addition, there can be moderate or extreme cravings for salt. The ability to combat stress and anxiety is a burden mainly upon these glands. Through the production of cortisol, the glands help fight inflammation. Furthermore, sugar is highly poisonous against them, as is alcohol.

    For the adrenal glands especially, the standard Western diet is destructive. While the brunt of the toxicity is suffered by this glandular system, the thyroid glands is also readily damaged by the noxious habits. Anyone brought up on a modern or Western diet is vulnerable for the development of adrenal collapse. This is especially true with the heavy or constant consumption of refined sugar. So, it would be expected that most thyroid types have at least a degree of adrenal component. It does help the thyroid gland heal and re-set to simultaneously support these glands. For more information see the adrenal self-test at www.ebodytype.com.

    There is no one easy approach to reversing the trend, so single supplement that typically suffices. Even so, the Body Shape Diet capsules are the closest example of such thoroughness. This plus the wild oregano extracts and B Complex might suffice in many cases.

THE HEALTH BENEFITS OF THYROID METABO...

There is the desire to get off the hormone drugs. This can be done in some cases through the supplement protocols listed here. Of particular importance is finding a replacement with the potentially toxic Synthroid. In addition to strong effects on the heart it also is a major cause of osteoporosis, which the take this truly wholesome, natural approach. So, to gain full function or the most that is possible it is crucial to take advantage of the wisdom of God. This will allow the healing miracles to occur. Every effort should be made to gain back the thyroid power that is so necessary for internal vitality. As a result, dramatic changes may result, including positive changes in the shape of the body and the reduction or elimination of fluid retention. Hormones have just that power. It is to either cause the decline of the body for worse, as in a deficiency, or restituting it to normal function.

With major changes in diet and proper supplementation so much can positively change. For the thyroid individual with this approach there can be a reduction of morning fatigue, overall exhaustion, cold sensitivity, chest congestion, memory weakness, depression, and far more. Let us gain these tremendous benefits, drug-free, following the truly natural way. Let us do so and thus relish in the benefit of the wisdom of non-synthetic therapy that will help to rebuild the function of the thyroid organ system. It is worth the effort, which is to have excellent function of this gland without the danger of medical and chemical intervention. It is all through the powers of divine nature. He would never leave us on this planet without providing the answers. Incredibly, these answers include how are body reacts to the imbalance by the shape of the torso, fat distribution, finger length, fluid retention sites, and tissue texture, all of which are revealed in this book. For confirmation see the testing systems at www.ebodytype.com.

Even without blood testing it is possible to find out where an individual stands and if there truly is a thyroid deficiency. That is the benefit of the Healthy Thyroid Metabolism plan.

Chapter Seven

Bibliography

Chaer, L., et al. 2015. Subclinical hypothyroidism and the risk for stroke events and fatal stroke: an individual participant data analysis. J. Clin Endocrin. Metab. 100:2181.

Ingram, C. 2004. Nutrition Tests for Better Health. Buffalo Grove, IL: Knowledge House Publishers.

Ingram, C. 2021. The Body Shape Code (formerly The Body Shape Diet). Lake Forest, IL: Knowledge House Publishers (available in Jan 2021)

Kim, T. K., et al. 2013. Effect of seasonal changes on transition between subclinical hypothyroid and euthyroid status. J. Clin. Endocrin. Metab. 98:3420.

Nanchen, D., et al. 2012. Subclinical thyroid dysfunction and the risk of heart failure in older persons at high cardiovascular risk. J. Clin. Endocrin. Metab. 97, issue 3.

Tepperman, J. 1977. Metabolic and Endocrine Physiology. Chicago: Yearbook Medical Publishers.

Williams, R.H. (ed). Textbook of Endocrinology. Philadelphia, PA: W.B. Saunders Co.

About the Author

Cass Ingram is a nutritional physician who received a B.S. in biology and chemistry from the University of Northern Iowa (1979) and a D.O. from Des Moines Osteopathic College (1984). During medical school, he took a keen interest in the field of endocrinology. He often said that the endocrine system is **responsible for nearly every cell, organ, and function in the body, and should not be overlooked in the treatment of illness**. He kept this in mind while treating patients. In the 1980's he started the Arlington Preventive Medical Center in Arlington Heights Illinois, which later became the American Center for Curative Medicine. Ingram was a pioneer in the holistic and preventive medical field. In the early 1990's he stumbled upon wild oregano on a trip to his mother's home country of Lebanon, and after extensive research, he wrote the book *The Cure is in the Cupboard*. He has written over 25 books on natural healing and has given answers and hope to millions through interviews on thousands of radio and TV shows, as well as on his podcast 'The Wilderness Doc'. His research and writing have led to countless nature based cures and discoveries. Cass Ingram presents hundreds of health tips and insights in his many books on health, nutrition, and disease prevention. He promotes the curative properties of wild medicinal foods and spice extracts. For more information see purelywild.cassingram.com.

Made in the USA
Columbia, SC
06 January 2025